The 3-D Library of the Human Body

THE LOWER LIMBS

LEARNING HOW WE USE OUR THIGHS, KNEES, LEGS, AND FEET

Jennifer Viegas

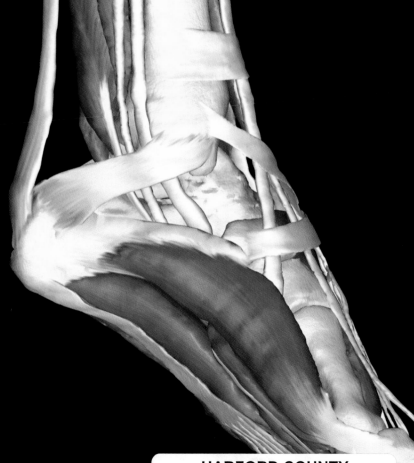

the rosen publishing group's
rosen
central

Editor's Note

The idea for the illustrations in this book originated in 1986 with the Vesalius Project at Colorado State University's Department of Anatomy and Neurobiology. There, a team of scientists and illustrators dreamed of turning conventional two-dimensional anatomical illustrations into three-dimensional computer images that could be rotated and viewed from any angle, for the benefit of students of medicine and biology. In 1988 this dream became the Visible Human Project™, under the sponsorship of the National Library of Medicine in Bethesda, Maryland. A grant was awarded to the University of Colorado School of Medicine, and in 1993 the first work of dissection and scanning began on the body of a Texas convict who had been executed by lethal injection. The process was repeated on the body of a Maryland woman who had died of a heart attack. Applying the latest techniques of computer graphics, the scientific team was able to create a series of three-dimensional digital images of the human body so beautiful and startlingly accurate that they seem more in the realm of art than science. On the computer screen, muscles, bones, and organs of the body can be turned and viewed from any angle, and layers of tissue can be electronically peeled away to reveal what lies underneath. In reproducing these digital images in two-dimensional print form, the editors at Rosen have tried to preserve the three-dimensional character of the work by showing organs of the body from different perspectives and using illustrations that progressively reveal deeper layers of anatomical structure.

Published in 2002 by The Rosen Publishing Group, Inc.
29 East 21st Street, New York, NY 10010

Digital anatomy images published by arrangement with Anatographica, LLC.
216 East 49th Street, New York, NY 10017

First Edition

Library of Congress Cataloging-in-Publication Data

Viegas, Jennifer.
The lower limbs: learning how we use our thighs, knees, legs, and feet / Jennifer Viegas. — 1st ed.
p. cm. — (The 3-D library of the human body)
Includes bibliographical references and index.
Summary: Discusses the anatomy and functions of the lower limbs and how we achieve coordinated and balanced movement with the muscles of our legs and feet.
ISBN 0-8239-3533-7
1. Leg—Juvenile literature. [1. Leg.]
I. Title. II. Series.
QM549 .V54 2001
611'.98—dc21

                                                                    2001003331

Manufactured in the United States of America

CONTENTS

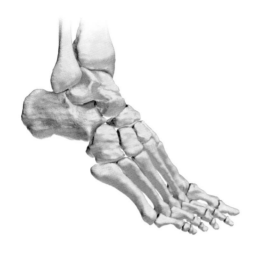

PREFACE
MYSTERIOUS
RAYS

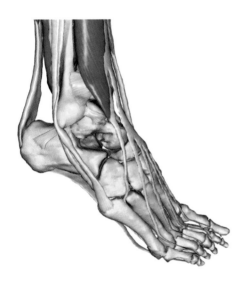

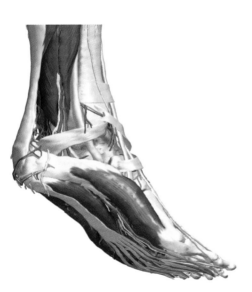

Our ability to understand the structure of the human body, and to diagnose and cure the illnesses of living patients, really began with the German physicist William Konrad Roentgen (1845–1923) and the mysterious rays he discovered in his laboratory on the winter evening of November 5, 1895.

Roentgen was never the best of students, not because of his lack of intelligence, but because of his maverick attitudes and his distrust of authority. In this respect, his early life parallels that of Albert Einstein (1879–1955). Like Einstein, he was asked to leave his school in Germany—he had ridiculed a teacher—before he had earned his degree, and he was only able to continue his education by moving to Switzerland and enrolling in the new Polytechnical Institute in Zurich. He finally obtained his doctorate in 1869 and became a professor of physics at the University of Würzburg in Bavaria, Germany.

Roentgen became very interested in the new phenomenon of cathode rays. Earlier scientists had noticed that when an electric current flowed across an open gap inside a glass tube from which the air had been removed, the tube began to fluoresce, or glow. Roentgen repeated this experiment, but he went a step further. He covered the glass tube with a layer of black cardboard so that no light could escape. When he turned on the current, he was amazed to discover that a sample of a barium compound on another table some distance from the cathode ray tube had begun to glow, even though no light had escaped from the glass tube. Some invisible ray, more powerful than light, had penetrated the black cardboard, traveled across the laboratory, and stimulated the fluorescent properties of the barium compound.

Roentgen named these strange rays X rays, because in science, "X" stands for the unknown, and Roentgen had no idea what these rays were. Soon Roentgen was exposing all sorts of materials to these rays and exploring their ability to penetrate some solid objects. Using photographic film, he produced a picture of the bones in his wife's hand. On January 23, 1896, he gave the first public demonstration of X rays, taking a picture of the bones in the hand of the Swiss anatomist Rudolf Kolliker.

Soon X rays were all the rage. Only four days after their discovery, American doctors used X rays to locate a bullet in a patient's leg. The earliest uses of X rays were in the diagnosis of tuberculosis and cancer. Unfortunately, it took several decades for people to realize that X rays could damage human tissue. Many doctors and researchers developed radiation burns and cancerous tumors, and more than 100 people died before the danger was recognized. In 1901, Roentgen received the prestigious Nobel prize for his discovery.

Today, X rays are still an essential tool for doctors, but we also have much more sophisticated techniques for seeing inside the human body without surgery. We have computerized axial tomography (CAT), positron emission tomography (PET), and magnetic resonance imaging (MRI). These techniques create three-dimensional images of internal organs by digitally assembling the data from hundreds of individual scans, and show degrees of detail impossible with X rays. Nevertheless, it all began with an unexpected flicker of light in a dark laboratory.

1
THE HIP AND THIGH

The lower limbs consist of the thighs, feet, and legs. Their main job is to bear the weight of the rest of the body and to allow for movement over distance, such as walking or running.

Some creatures get by without any lower limbs. Worms and snakes, for example, are able to wiggle and slither quite fast along the ground. Slithering has its limits, though. The muscles of a snake must have something to push against in order for movement to occur. A snake placed on a completely smooth surface, like a clean plate of glass, cannot slither.

Other animals and insects have four, six, eight, or even more legs to carry them around. More legs give animals, like horses and dogs, good support and balance. A cheetah, the fastest land animal, can run at a speed of seventy-five miles per hour, or ten miles over the speed limit allowed for cars on most U.S. highways.

Unlike cheetahs, people have only two legs. While humans cannot run as fast as most four-legged animals, having two legs frees the hands and allows for a variety of movements, from swimming to climbing trees. Standing and moving with two legs is difficult for most creatures. Think of watching dogs, chimpanzees, or gorillas attempting to walk on two limbs. However, the lower limbs of humans, which begin at the hip, allow people to stand and move easily with their two legs.

The Hip

The hipbone, also called the pelvis, holds the hips and legs in place and also cradles the bladder, the sac that holds liquid waste from the body. The bones that look like giant mouse ears at the top form the ilium, or pelvic girdle. The ilium is what can be felt when the hands are placed on the hips. The upside-down triangle in the middle consists of the sacrum and coccyx, or tailbone. These are several vertebrae that are

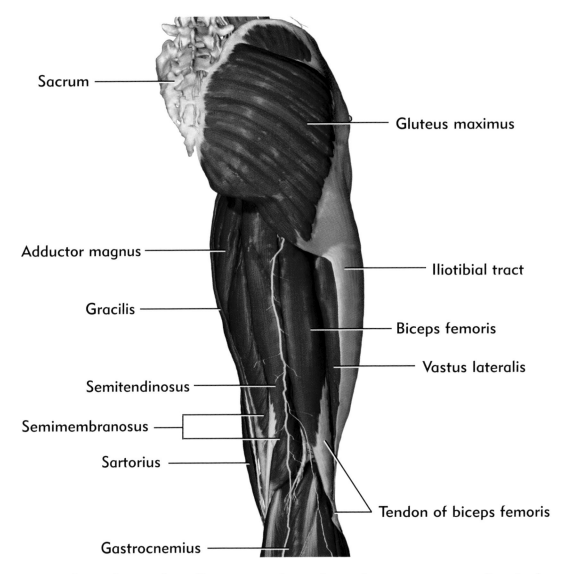

Sacrum

Gluteus maximus

Adductor magnus

Iliotibial tract

Gracilis

Biceps femoris

Vastus lateralis

Semitendinosus

Semimembranosus

Sartorius

Tendon of biceps femoris

Gastrocnemius

The biceps femoris, semitendinosus, and semimembranosus are collectively known as the hamstring.

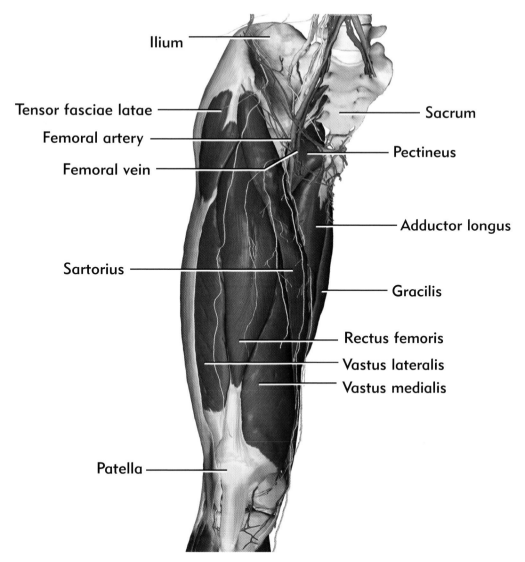

Ilium

Tensor fasciae latae

Femoral artery

Femoral vein

Sartorius

Patella

Sacrum

Pectineus

Adductor longus

Gracilis

Rectus femoris

Vastus lateralis

Vastus medialis

An anterior (front) view of the thigh. The bones of the lower limbs are thicker and the muscles are larger and stronger than those of the upper limbs.

fused together. Vertebrae, in turn, are small rings of bone that protect the spinal cord and form the backbone. Bend your back slightly and you can feel the vertebrae along your spine.

The legs are attached to the hip in a socket called the acetabulum. The acetabula (plural for acetabulum) lie at opposite ends of the hipbone and face outward. This improves balance and range of movement. Imagine if the acetabula were stuck together at the front of the hip. People would be forced to take tiny steps, leaning backward for balance! Each acetabulum has an inward curve that accommodates the ball-shaped end of the femur, or thighbone. Together, the round head of the femur and the acetabulum create what is known as a ball-and-socket joint.

Joints

Joints are places where two bones meet. The body has many joints. For example, take a look at your finger. Each finger has three joints. One is near where the knuckle meets the hand and the other two joints are where the finger bends. Feel how these joints define separate bones in a finger.

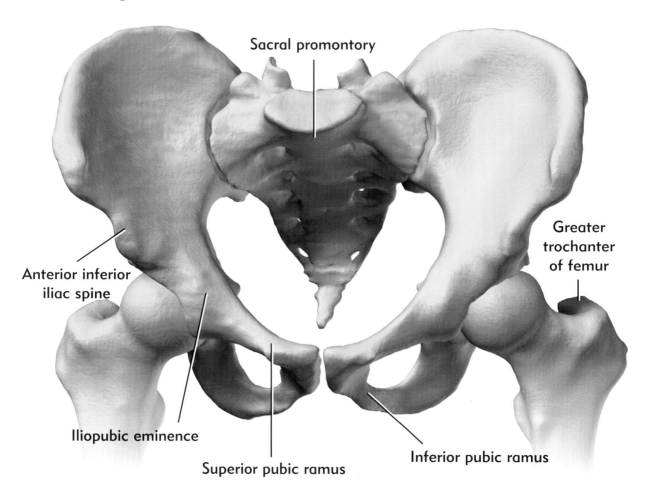

Sacral promontory

Anterior inferior
iliac spine

Greater
trochanter
of femur

Iliopubic eminence

Superior pubic ramus

Inferior pubic ramus

In addition to supporting and protecting the pelvic organs, the pelvic bone provides a large surface for the attachment of the trunk and leg muscles.

There are three main types of joints in the body: moveable ones, called synovial joints; fixed ones, called fibrous joints; and cartilaginous joints, places where bone meets with cartilage, a flexible, gristle-like material. Synovial refers to a membrane, or thin sheet of tissue, that lines certain joints. This tissue releases synovial fluid, which is a slippery substance that makes moving easier. Synovial fluid is similar to the oil used to repair a squeaky door with a tight hinge.

Synovial joints can be divided into different types, depending on how they move and work. The ball-and-socket joint in the pelvis is one such type. It allows for a full range of movement. Thanks to this kind of joint in the pelvis, people can swing their legs around in a circle. Keep this in mind when watching people twist and turn their legs while playing sports, such as football and basketball, or while dancing and skating. With every move of the upper leg, the circular top of the femur bone rotates in the ball-

Spinal nerves descending through the pelvic area

and-socket joint. The synovial fluid ensures that such movements are smooth and without friction, or rubbing, which can cause damage.

External iliac artery

Femoral artery

Femoral vein

Nerves

Nerves are bundles of special tissue that carry messages to and from the brain. The spinal cord at the center of the back, which is protected by the vertebrae, serves as a collection center for nerves within the body. All nerves originate at the spinal cord and branch out to every part of the body, from the tips of the fingers to the bottoms of the feet. Around the hip area, nerves look like large sprigs of grass sprouting from the spine.

Through electrical impulses that release neurotransmitter chemicals, nerves can control movement. In a chain reaction, individual nerve cells, called neurons, pass electrical impulses to each other until the contained message reaches its destination. For example, lift a leg now. In that split second, the brain sends a message down through the spinal cord and to the leg, with countless neuron exchanges occurring along the way. At the leg, the neurons instruct muscles there to move.

This image reveals the main arteries and veins of the pelvic and thigh area.

The Thigh

The area between the hip and knee is the thigh. Most animals with legs, including humans, have thighs. In fact, ham and leg of lamb are cuts of meat that come from the thighs of pigs and lambs. Thighs are thick, fleshy, and muscular. Thigh muscles are needed to support and move the body.

Muscles

Muscles are strong and powerful tissues that are responsible for all body movements. When stimulated by nerves, muscles contract, or shorten and become tighter, which pulls bones closer together. An important point to remember is that muscles can pull, but they cannot push. This means that different muscles are required for varying movements.

The gluteus meteus muscle at each pelvic ball-and-socket joint controls the turning, rotating, and extending of the thigh. Just behind the gluteus meteus is the gluteus maximus. This big muscle aids the gluteus meteus in extending and rotating the

The main nerves of the lower limbs run down the femur, or thighbone.

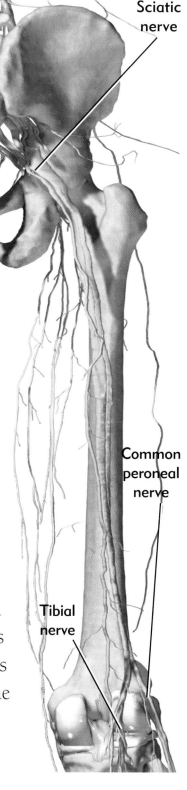

Sciatic nerve

Common peroneal nerve

Tibial nerve

Measure Thigh Muscle Strength

All healthy individuals have strong thigh muscles that carry the weight of the body and move the legs. Here is a fun way to measure thigh muscle strength. With permission, take a bathroom scale, preferably one that is no longer needed to measure weight, and place it between the knees. Now, squeeze as hard as possible. Have someone write down the scale reading. The number is a measurement of how strong the inner thigh muscles are. Exercise can strengthen muscles, so try to increase the number over time by exercising the thigh and leg muscles regularly.

thigh. It also braces the knee. The sartorius muscle, which wraps around the front of the thigh, is the longest muscle in the body. It flexes and rotates the thigh and leg. Two of the main muscles at the front of the thigh are the rectus femoris and the vastus lateralis.

Like big computer cables, muscles are made out of thick bands that contain smaller fibers. Within each muscle fiber—about the size of a strand of hair—are even smaller myofibrils. These, in turn, contain ultra tiny threads, called myosin and actin filaments, that interact and allow for muscle contraction and relaxation. While the process is complex, basically the filaments move closer together during contraction, causing the muscle to pull. During relaxation, the filaments move farther apart, and the muscle relaxes.

2
THE THIGH AND KNEE

Underneath the skin of the thigh, the thigh muscles can be seen as thick, fleshy strands. If the leg were lifted, these strands would contract, causing the leg to move in a certain direction, depending on which muscle was used. Notice the white bands attached to the ends of the thigh muscles. These are tendons.

Tendons

Tendons connect muscles to bones. Whenever a muscle contracts, the tendon pulls on a bone, which allows for movement. While the muscle areas of the thigh contain several nerve endings and are supplied with a lot of blood, the tendons are, for the most part, inactive. They are like very strong puppet strings. To control a puppet, someone must tug, or stretch and shorten, the string, causing the attached puppet to move. In the case of tendons, muscles stretch and shorten. The attached tendons then respond to this activity by moving. Bones at the end are like puppets. They have no motion by themselves, but simply react to muscle contractions transmitted through tendons.

Tendons, also sometimes called sinews, are made up of very strong connective tissue. Although tendons are located in the body and not on its surface, it is possible to feel what a tendon is like. Place a hand at the back of your knee and swing your lower leg back and forth. The

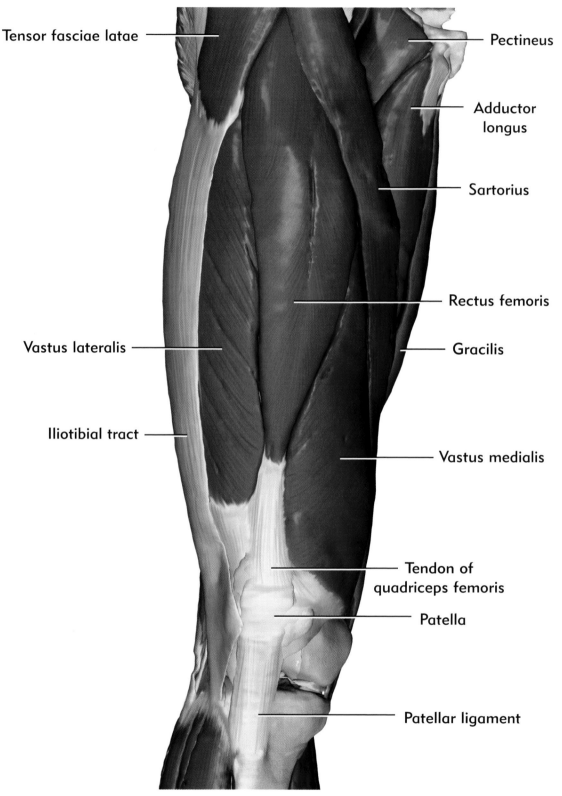

Tensor fasciae latae

Pectineus

Adductor longus

Sartorius

Rectus femoris

Vastus lateralis

Gracilis

Iliotibial tract

Vastus medialis

Tendon of quadriceps femoris

Patella

Patellar ligament

The three muscles that make up the powerful quadriceps femoris flex the thigh at the hip and extend the limb at the knee.

stretching and relaxing sensation is actually the hamstring tendon, connected to the hamstring muscles of the thigh, moving the lower leg bones back and forth.

The Knee

The knee is the biggest joint in the body. It marks the separation between the bone of the upper thigh, the femur, and the bones of the lower leg, the tibia and the smaller fibula next to it. This is one tough joint! Consider a door joint, for example. Imagine what would happen to the door if it were slammed open and shut all day. At the very least, the joint would require constant maintenance. Over time it would probably have to be repaired or replaced.

Knees take this kind of abuse every day. Think of how many times the knees must bend. They bend when a person sits, walks, kicks, runs, and even sleeps. Because of all of the potential wear and tear, knees have a more complex construction than other joints.

In the same way that the hipbone has grooves where it meets the thighbone, the top of the tibia is slightly concave, or cup-shaped, where it meets the femur. Given all of the movement in this region, these two bones could grind against each other without protection. Cartilage takes care of this by forming a protective surface at the knee where the leg bones meet.

Cartilage

Cartilage is a tough, yet flexible, part of the body that is mostly found in joints, such as the knee, and other places where flexibility is essential. Most of the nose and ears are cartilage, which is why these areas respond easily to touch and motion, such as when the nostrils are pinched together or when the ears move when a sweater or shirt is pulled over them.

Cartilage is constructed like a net with cells and fibers running through it. These fibers are made from proteins called collagen and elastin. Manufacturers of cosmetics often refer to these terms because the protein fibers, also found in skin, can degrade with age and are associated with wrinkle formation. Collagen also is what mostly makes the dark meat in chicken different than the white meat. Just as humans have a lot of collagen in the leg cartilage, birds also have it in their wings and legs.

In images of the knee, cartilage can be seen between the thigh and calf bones. The top disk of cartilage is called the medial meniscus, while the one that rests over the tibia is called the lateral meniscus. Together they are called menisci. The knee can function without the protection of cartilage, but not always as smoothly. Athletes often suffer torn cartilage, and the cartilage has to be removed. Sometimes this can lead to arthritis and other problems later in life.

Synovial fluid surrounds the cartilage and joint area of the knee. "Synovial" comes from the Greek word for "egg white," which this fluid somewhat resembles. In addition to the oil-like synovial lubricant, two other sacs of fluid, called bursae, rest between the femur and tibia. The bursae are like little cushions that relieve stress and strain on the joint. Ligaments are in the middle of the joint too, and also lie on either side of the knee.

Ligaments

Ligaments are similar to tendons, except that they link bones to other bones and are made of more flexible tissue. Without ligaments, bones in the body would easily become dislocated, like a model airplane that was not glued together properly. While ligaments hold bones together, they also allow for movement. Try walking without bending the knees. It is awkward and not easy. The ligaments in the knee hold the bones

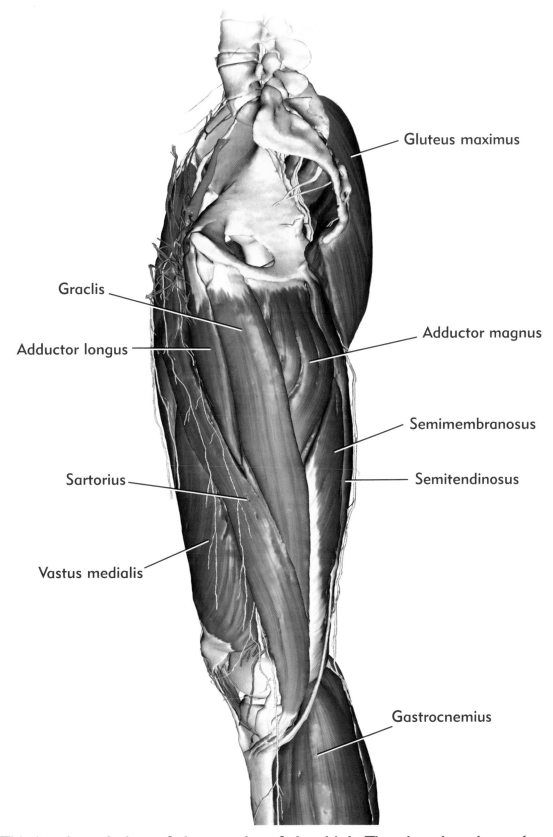

Gluteus maximus

Graclis

Adductor longus

Adductor magnus

Semimembranosus

Semitendinosus

Sartorius

Vastus medialis

Gastrocnemius

This is a lateral view of the muscles of the thigh. The gluteal, or buttock, muscles extend the hip and are very important for running and climbing.

Femur

Patella

Tibia

of the leg together, but still allow the knee joint to bend. The posterior cruciate ligament and anterior cruciate ligament hold the knee together at the joint, while the tibia collateral ligament at the front of the knee and the fibular collateral ligament at the back keep the legs straight and help to prevent the knee from bending backwards.

The kneecap is like a built-in kneepad. It is actually a disk-shaped bone, called the patella. Tendons in the body do not usually have bones, but the patella is an exception, as it is part of the tendon of the quadriceps muscle in the thigh. The patella protects this tendon from wearing down due to the joint bending.

The joint at the knee is called a hinge joint. Unlike the ball-and-socket joint at the hips, which allows for a full range of movement, the knee can only move back and forth. The knee bends in the same way that the pages of a book open and close. The knee does not have to swing around in a circle, as the entire leg can move the knee along with it. Also, the

The bones of the femur and the tibia meet at the kneecap.

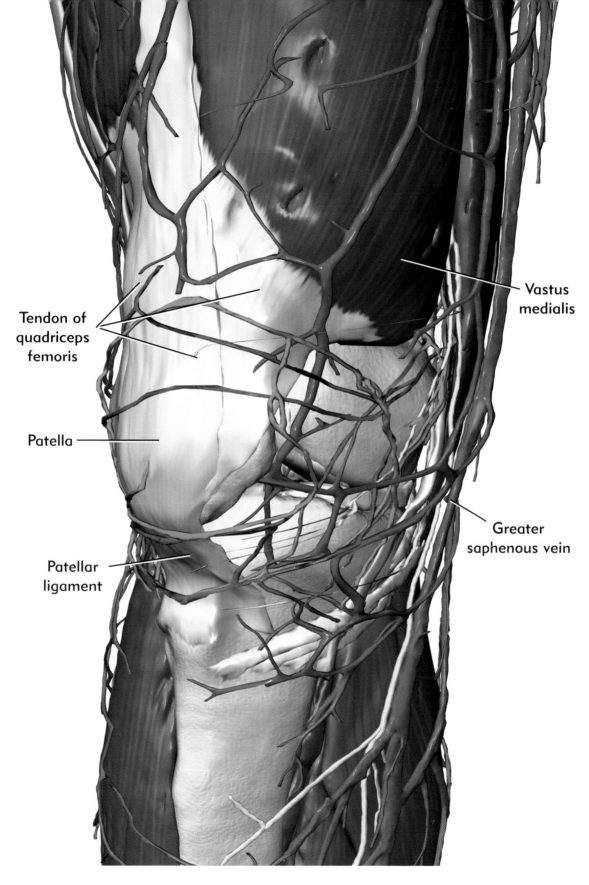

Tendon of
quadriceps
femoris

Vastus
medialis

Patella

Greater
saphenous vein

Patellar
ligament

This image reveals the muscles and blood vessels of the knee.

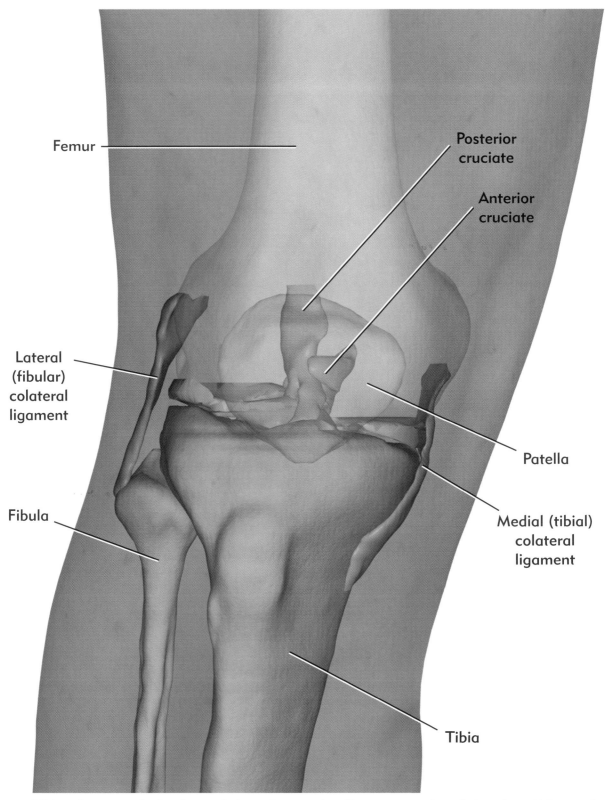

Femur

Posterior
cruciate

Anterior
cruciate

Lateral
(fibular)
colateral
ligament

Patella

Fibula

Medial (tibial)
colateral
ligament

Tibia

This picture of the knee joint shows the ligaments that join the tibia and the femur.

Knee-Jerk Reflex

Reflexes are automatic reactions that the body performs to protect itself. One of the most well known is called the knee-jerk reflex. Doctors often test this reflex to see how well a patient's muscles and nerves are working. They do this by tapping the tendon below the kneecap. Nerves in the tendon travel to the spinal cord, which sends a signal to the muscles at the front of the thigh to contract, causing the knee to jerk forward. The patient becomes aware of the response later, after a message has had time to travel to the brain.

hinge mechanism allows the knees to lock in place so that a person can stand with little effort. Standing up straight with both feet on the ground is not only best for the spine, but it also puts less strain on the knees.

As the largest and heaviest joint, the knee is also the body's most vulnerable one. Although well protected by cartilage, synovial fluid, the bursae, and ligaments, the knee should still be guarded during periods of active use, such as when playing football or rollerblading, with kneepads or some other form of protection. Think of all of the great sports stars that have had to curtail their careers due to knee problems. The knee is injured more than any other joint, but proper care can help to prevent it from sustaining damage.

3
THE LEG, CALF, AND SHIN

Below the knee and above the foot are the calf and shin. The calf forms the back of the lower leg, and the shin refers to the front part of the lower leg. Bones provide structure to this area, as well as to the entire leg. The femur in the thigh is the biggest, longest, and heaviest bone in the whole body. The tibia, under the knee, is the second-largest bone. The fibula, next to the tibia, is large too, but doesn't compare in size to the other major leg bones. The leg bones are big because they have to support both themselves and the upper body.

These three bones, along with the other 203 bones in the body, have a unique structure that makes them, pound for pound, more sturdy and strong than concrete, wood, and even steel. Steel girders hold up giant buildings, including skyscrapers, so imagine how strong human bones are. While the inner structure of bones can slightly vary, depending on where the bones are located, the basic components remain the same.

Before birth, the bones of a baby in the womb are made of flexible cartilage. At birth, the cartilage has developed into hard bone. While bones are strong, they are light and not solid. The exterior is often referred to as hard bone. It is actually a tough substance made up of numerous cells. The cells, or the building blocks of all living things, link together to form rings around small holes that can be detected under a microscope. The holes allow blood to pass through and nourish the bone.

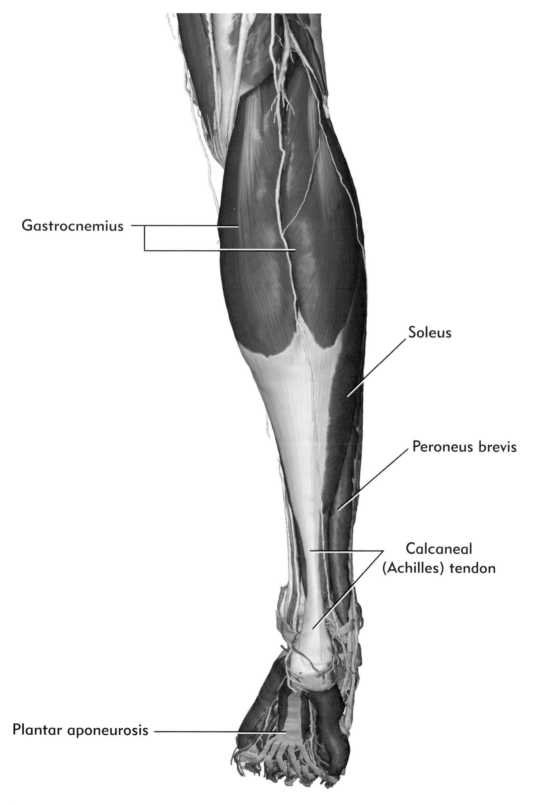

Gastrocnemius

Soleus

Peroneus brevis

Calcaneal
(Achilles) tendon

Plantar aponeurosis

This is a posterior, or rear, view of the muscles of the calf. The muscles of the lower leg move the foot and the toes.

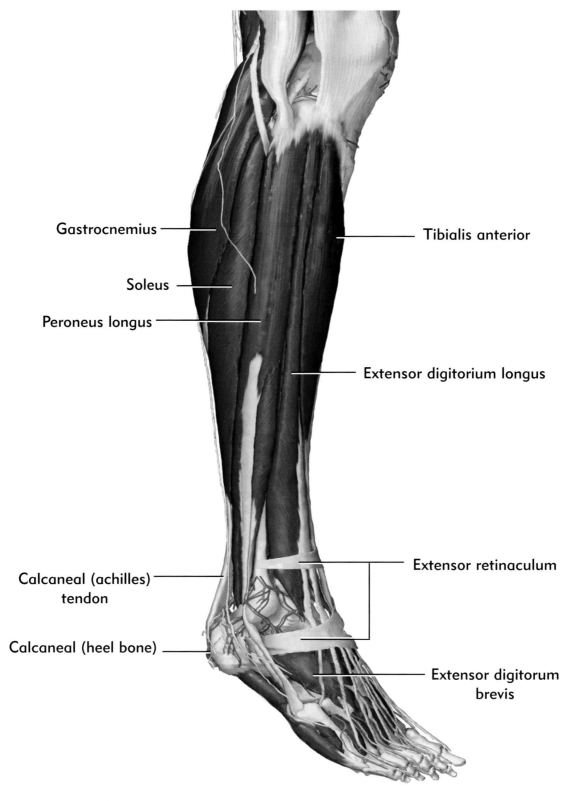

Gastrocnemius

Soleus

Peroneus longus

Tibialis anterior

Extensor digitorium longus

Calcaneal (achilles) tendon

Calcaneal (heel bone)

Extensor retinaculum

Extensor digitorum brevis

With the ankle as a pivot, the muscles of the lower leg provide the force to push the feet off the ground during walking and running.

Blood cells are created in the honeycomb-like centers of many bones. There, marrow, a material similar to jelly, falls into two different types: red and yellow. Red marrow makes red blood cells, which help to distribute oxygen throughout the body. Red marrow also produces germ-fighting white blood cells and platelets, which help blood to clot. Yellow marrow, on the other hand, stores fat and distributes it around the body as needed.

Bones keep growing until about the time a person reaches the age of twenty. That is one reason why people continue to get taller through their teens. Bones also rejuvenate themselves, up until the age of thirty-five or so, creating new bone to replace older, damaged spots. After thirty-five, however, this repair process slows down.

Bones store minerals, such as calcium. Like fat from yellow marrow, bones release the minerals when they are needed by other parts of the body. As a person ages, a lot of the minerals and collagen have already left the bone, which is why older people sometimes suffer from brittle bones and are vulnerable to bone fractures. It is often necessary for such individuals to take calcium supplements, to help deter this aging process.

Despite the fact that they can be broken, bones can often heal themselves. The healing process begins almost immediately. About an hour after a break, blood oozes out of the broken ends to form a clot. Approximately two days later, bone cells called fibroblasts and osteoblasts string together, forming a loose connection between the broken ends. Gradually, other cells fill in the open spaces and the bone hardens. After about three months, most broken bones have fully mended. To help this happen, doctors often put a cast over the affected area, which holds the bones in place and makes sure the broken parts join together properly.

The thigh muscles are connected to bones in the lower leg. Major muscles of the shin area at the front of the lower leg include the peroneus

What Exercise Does to Leg Muscles

Weight lifters and bodybuilders often have huge leg muscles that bulge and ripple underneath the skin. Interestingly enough, these individuals have the same number of muscle fibers as a couch potato who rarely exercises. Well-trained athletes, however, have larger muscle fibers that contain more actin and myosin. They also develop more connective tissue and have stronger bones and tendons, which is why they can lift heavy objects. While weight lifting may not be for everyone, regular exercise is important for maintaining the health of muscles, keeping body fat to a minimum, and ensuring strong legs for years to come.

longus muscle, which aids in walking, the tibialis anterior muscle, which moves the foot up, and the soleus muscle, which flexes the foot down. A major muscle of the calf area at the back of the lower leg is the gastroc-nemius muscle. Like the soleus muscle, it helps to flex the foot into a downward position. It also can flex the entire leg.

A side view of the lower leg reveals the Achilles tendon, also sometimes called the Achilles' heel. It looks like a slender white triangle that runs from the back of the leg to the back of the foot. As with all tendons, the job of the Achilles tendon is to link muscle to bone. Note how it links the large gastrocnemius muscle to bone in the foot.

The Achilles tendon is the strongest tendon in the entire body. Because it is so big and strong, this tendon can be easily felt. Try to feel it now, by placing a hand at the calf where your leg meets your foot. Now, point the toes of that foot and bend the foot into an upward position. The tighten-ing sensation is the tendon pulling on the foot bone.

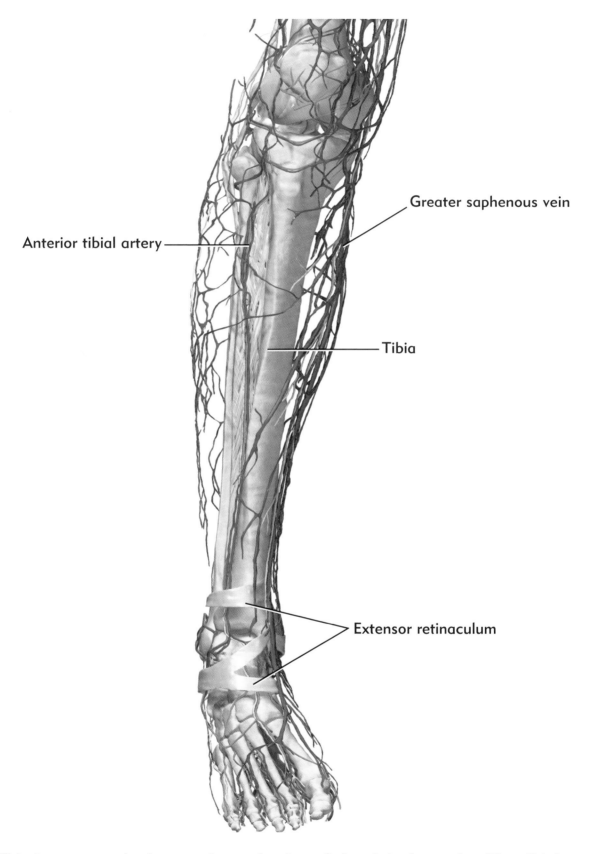

Greater saphenous vein

Anterior tibial artery

Tibia

Extensor retinaculum

This image reveals the arteries and veins of the right lower leg. The tibial arteries supply blood to the anterior and posterior muscles of the legs.

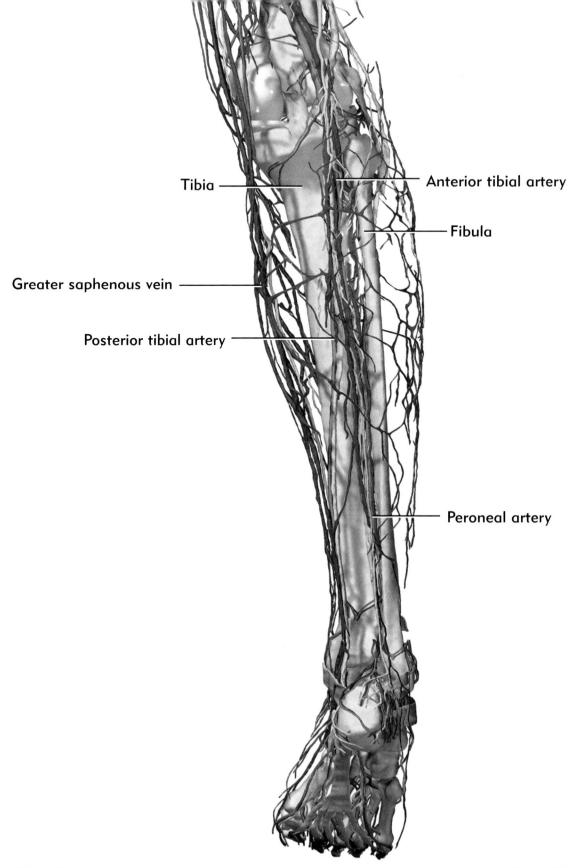

Tibia

Anterior tibial artery

Fibula

Greater saphenous vein

Posterior tibial artery

Peroneal artery

This illustration shows the arteries and veins of the left lower leg. The tibial arteries receive blood from the femoral artery in the thigh.

The Achilles tendon is named after Achilles, a warrior in Greek mythology. According to this legend, Achilles' mother tried to make him immortal by dipping him into a sacred river. Unfortunately, she held him by the heel, which never touched the water, so the heel did not receive any special powers. It remained vulnerable. Similarly, the Achilles tendon does not have the same protection the patella gives the tendon in front of the thigh. As a result, this tendon is at risk from damage caused by strenuous exertion or from shoes that do not fit properly.

Surrounding the Achilles tendon and other internal parts of the legs are blood vessels, or tubes that move blood through the body. There are two types of blood vessels: arteries and veins. Arteries carry blood away from the heart and veins carry blood to the heart. Blood travels along arteries like a car on a highway, making stops to deliver oxygen, nutrients, and other essential things that help to sustain and fuel the legs. That is one reason why the heart rate of a person who is running increases. The leg muscles need more oxygen and fuel, so the heart pumps harder to increase the blood supply. Veins then pick up low-oxygen blood that needs reenergizing and deliver it back to the heart, which pumps the blood into the lungs for an oxygen fill-up.

There are many arteries and veins in the legs, each with its own name. The iliac arteries and veins, for example, take care of blood deliveries and pickups from the pelvic region to the thighs. Originating near the knees, femoral arteries and veins control blood that is transported through the lower legs.

Nerves originating from the spine also branch out within the legs. Major leg nerves include the sciatic nerves, which run through the hipbone and into the thighs; the femoral nerves, which, like the femoral arteries and veins, run down the femurs and into the lower legs; and the sural nerves, which carry messages to the feet.

4
THE FEET

Consider the size of the feet in relation to the size of the rest of the body. A foot is often less than half as big as a person's arm and is not nearly as thick and muscular as the thigh, yet the feet carry the weight of the entire body. Most people know about how to dress the foot with the latest high-tech sports shoes and fashionable footwear, but consider the incredible structure of the feet themselves.

The area where a lower leg meets a foot is full of muscle endings and tendons. The reason for so many tendons is that, while the foot contains muscles, most of the muscles that control foot movement are in the legs. This allows the feet to move freely without being weighed down by huge muscles. Imagine, for example, if the thigh muscles were in the foot. People would clomp around in awkward, heavy steps. Because there are so many tendons in the foot, the tendons are enclosed in sheaths.

Tendon Sheaths

Tendon sheaths in the foot look a bit like shoehorns. They are located where the front part of the foot curves to form the shin. The job of tendon sheaths is to protect the many tendons of the foot from sustaining damage due to friction and abrasion. The sheaths consist of

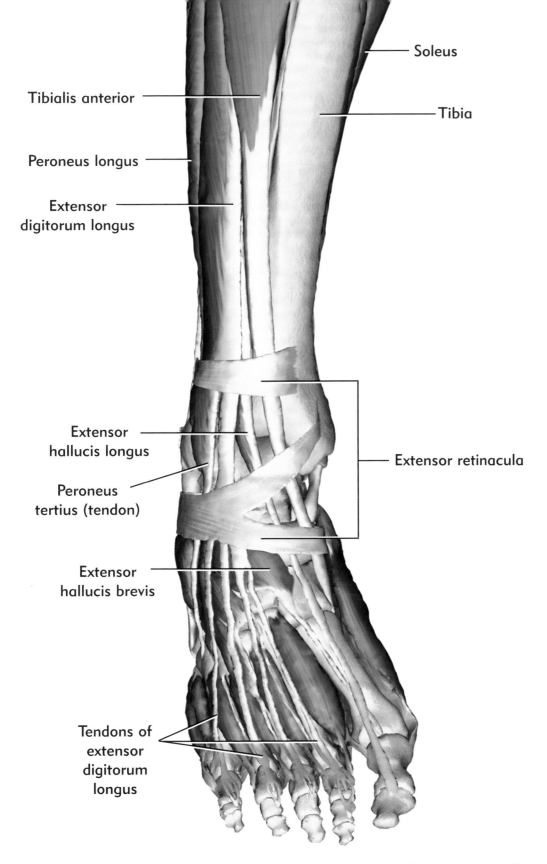

Soleus

Tibialis anterior

Tibia

Peroneus longus

Extensor
digitorum longus

Extensor
hallucis longus

Extensor retinacula

Peroneus
tertius (tendon)

Extensor
hallucis brevis

Tendons of
extensor
digitorum
longus

The muscles and cartilage of the foot are shown here. The foot acts like a
lever to push the leg off of the ground when we walk, run, and jump.

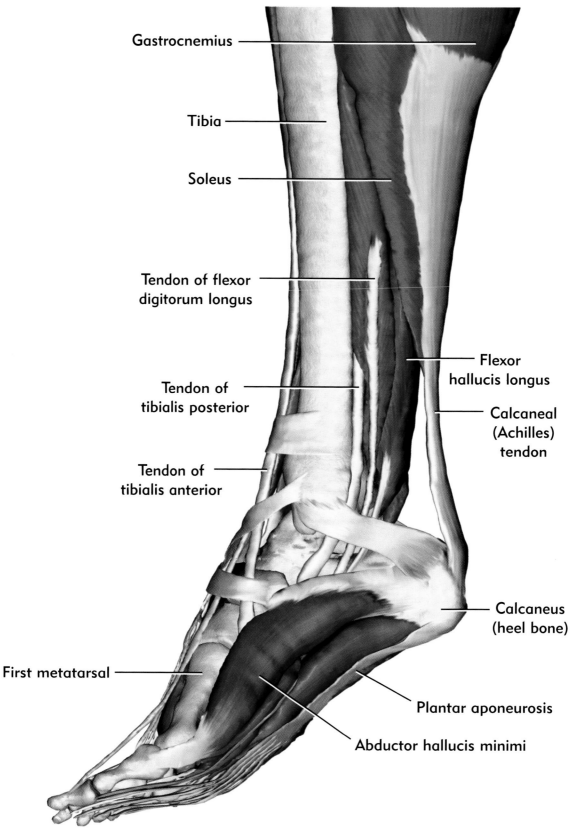

Gastrocnemius

Tibia

Soleus

Tendon of flexor
digitorum longus

Tendon of
tibialis posterior

Tendon of
tibialis anterior

First metatarsal

Flexor
hallucis longus

Calcaneal
(Achilles)
tendon

Calcaneus
(heel bone)

Plantar aponeurosis

Abductor hallucis minimi

This is a medial view of the foot and ankle. The muscles of the calf end in strong tendons.

a double layer of tissue. The space between the layers, where the tendons lie, is filled with lubricating fluid. The fluid allows the tendons within the sheath to slide back and forth with ease. Given all of the abuse feet take, the tendon sheaths come in handy. For example, think of playing soccer or football. With every kick, the tendons must withstand the forceful blow.

Just as athletes sometimes wrap parts of the body with tape, the feet are bound together by broad ligaments. These look like masking tape wound around where the lower leg meets the ankle. These ligaments help to hold the foot's many tendons in place. The fleshy parts under the tendons in the foot consist of skeletal muscles. These give the foot its shape. The skeletal muscles also pull on the tendons at the tip of the foot, which moves the toes.

When a Foot Falls Asleep

When a foot is held in an awkward position for a long time it can "fall asleep." This often occurs when a person sits on a foot for too long. A foot that is asleep may feel numb. That is because too much pressure has blocked sensory nerves. The nerves can no longer send messages to the spine and into the brain, so the foot loses feeling. When the individual stands up and shakes the affected foot around, the nerves gradually recover. During this time, the person will likely feel a tingling sensation as the nerves regain the ability to send and receive messages.

Toes

The toes on each foot are designed to aid in walking. During a zoo visit, check out what similar digits look like on the feet and legs of chimpanzees and birds. The chimp equivalent of toes actually look more like fingers, which is one reason why chimps can climb better than humans. Bird legs often have thin sticklike ends, which provide support but are not as good for walking.

Humans have five toes on each foot. The scientific name for the big toe is the hallux. Next to it is the second toe, followed by the third, fourth, and fifth, or little, toe. The big toe has its own muscles, which is why it can move around in several directions. Try moving a big toe now. Now try to move each of the three middle toes by themselves. What happens? The reason it is not possible for the three middle toes to move individually is because they share the same muscles. The little toe, like the big toe, has its own muscles. It, however, has a more limited range of movement.

The toenails cover the tops of the ends of the toes. In the early years of human evolution, people walked barefoot and the toenails wore down by themselves. Now they require regular trimming. The reason this does not hurt is because the nails themselves are dead. Nails are attached to the toes by a root, which does contain living cells.

Bones in the feet are soft compared to those of the thigh and lower leg. This provides greater flexibility and aids in walking. At the top of the foot, the tibia and fibula bones of the lower leg fit into the talus. The tibia and fibula bulge out on either side, forming the medial malleolus and the lateral malleolus. These create the ankle (they can be felt with the fingers).

Below the talus is a large bone called the calcaneus. It forms the heel of the foot. Tarsal bones are the relatively short bones in front of the talus and calcaneus. The metatarsals are longer and are arranged in front of the tarsals. Finally, the toes get their structure from phalange bones.

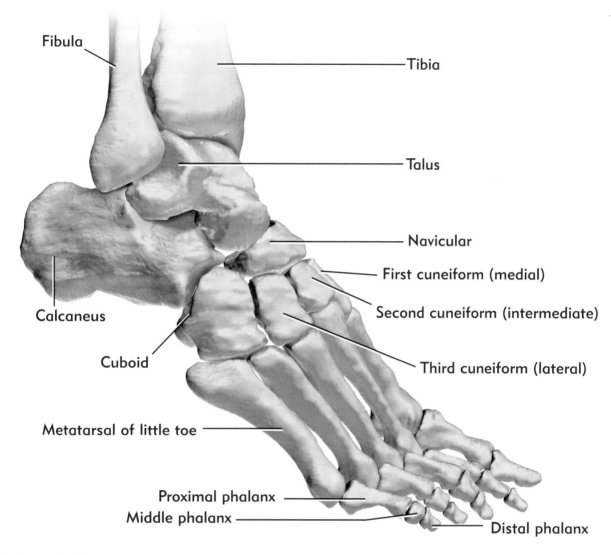

A lateral view of the bones of the foot. The foot provides a flexible and resilient base to support the weight of the body.

Balance, Walking, and Running

Three functions performed by the feet are walking, running, and maintaining balance. Balancing the body on two legs requires a bit of work. This skill comes naturally, for the most part, yet the legs are constantly sending messages to the brain as to what is the best way to stay balanced. Sensory nerves in the feet, for example, let the brain know what kind of surface the feet have to adapt to, whether it is a smooth pavement or a sandy beach. These senses can be fooled, though. Try standing barefoot on a pillow with both arms stretched outward for balance. Now, with a friend nearby to help, place a blindfold over your eyes, lift one leg, and place your arms to the sides. The friend may have to provide balance, as the foot touching the pillow will struggle to keep the body standing upright.

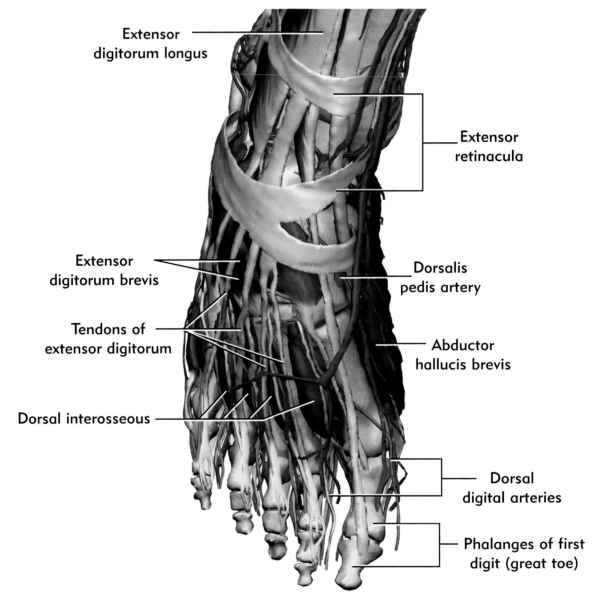

Extensor digitorum longus

Extensor retinacula

Extensor digitorum brevis

Dorsalis pedis artery

Tendons of extensor digitorum

Abductor hallucis brevis

Dorsal interosseous

Dorsal digital arteries

Phalanges of first digit (great toe)

These are the muscles and blood vessels of the foot. The small muscles in the foot constantly adjust our balance.

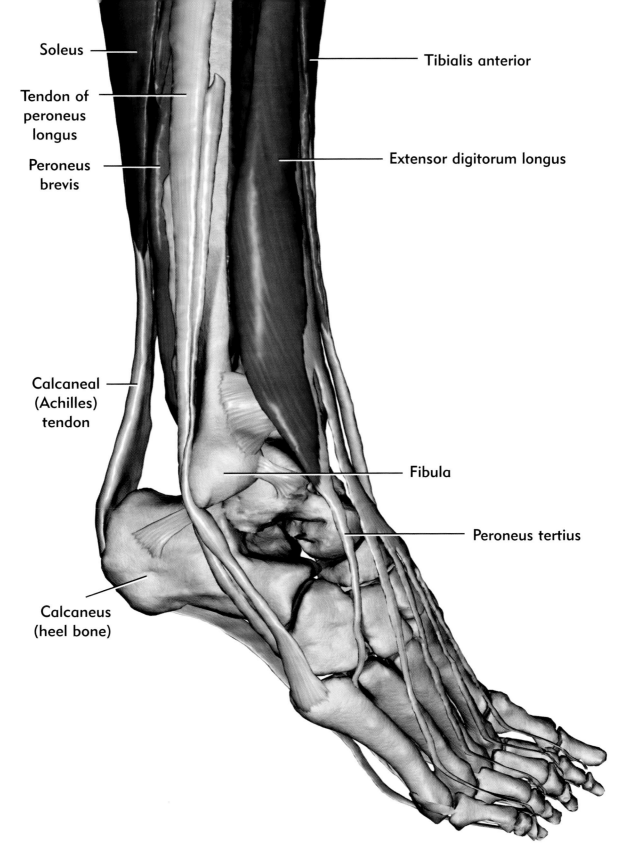

Soleus

Tendon of peroneus longus

Peroneus brevis

Calcaneal (Achilles) tendon

Calcaneus (heel bone)

Tibialis anterior

Extensor digitorum longus

Fibula

Peroneus tertius

The foot is adapted for stability and weight-bearing capacity, but is also surprisingly flexible.

Walking is yet another function performed by the feet and legs that requires skill. Babies cannot walk when they are born. They have to learn how to coordinate the parts of the body. Coordination is like programming a computer. The brain has to fine-tune the muscles and nerves so that they will work together in unison. When a baby takes its first steps, it truly is a special moment, because at that point, he or she has coordinated the movements necessary for walking.

Running requires a more advanced form of coordination and a great deal of footwork. As each foot pounds to the ground, the weight of the entire body descends down from the tibia and into the talus. That is one reason why good running shoes provide ample talus, or ankle, support. The weight then pushes forward to the tarsals and metatarsals before it moves backward to the calcaneus. With such a pounding, it becomes evident why so many muscles, tendons, bones, and ligaments are needed in the feet.

Though they are learned skills, walking and running are fairly basic functions. Using the same learning process, people can perform other incredible feats with their feet. Think of track and field athletes who perform long jumps and leap over hurdles. Gymnasts can learn to walk gracefully on a thin bar. Basketball players can dunk the ball with a split second twist and jump. Ballet dancers can even balance their entire body on their toes. With practice, the limits of foot and leg coordination are virtually endless.

GLOSSARY

Achilles tendon Long tendon that runs from the calf to the heel of the foot.

actin Protein that, along with another protein, myosin, is responsible for muscle contraction.

ball-and-socket joint Joint, such as where the acetabulum in the hip meets the femur bone of the thigh, that allows for full rotational movement.

bone Multilayered hard tissue made primarily of collagen fibers and minerals that provides support and structure to the body.

calf Back part of the lower leg.

cartilage More flexible than bone, cartilage is a protective tissue found in the nose, ears, and around the ends of bones at joints.

collagen Tough protein found in skin, cartilage, and bone.

contract Shortening and tightening of muscles, which causes them to pull up bones attached by tendons.

femur This longest and heaviest bone of the body begins at the hip and forms the upper part of the knee joint.

fibula Bone located in the lower leg that begins at the lower part of the knee joint and ends at the foot.

hinge joint Joint that allows for back and forth movement, such as the hinge joint at the knee.

joint Place where two or more bones meet.

ligament Firm, bandlike tissue that holds bones together at joints.

marrow Soft material in the center of bones.

muscle Strong tissues that give bones and the rest of the body movement.

nerve Cylindrical fibers that originate from the spinal cord and carry messages to and from the brain.

neuron Nerve cells, or building blocks, that make up nerves.

patella Disk of bone, commonly referred to as the kneecap, that protects the tendon at the front of the knee joint.

reflex Involuntary movement performed by the body, usually to protect itself, as exemplified by the knee-jerk reflex.

shin   Front part of the lower leg.

synovial fluid   Oil-like liquid that lubricates certain joints, such as those found at the hip and knee.

talus   Commonly called the anklebone, the talus is located just above the heel in the foot.

tendon   Fibrous band of tissue that connects muscle to bone.

tendon sheath   Double-layered tissue that protects tendons, such as those located in the feet.

tibia   This second largest bone of the body begins at the lower part of the knee joint and ends at the foot.

FOR MORE INFORMATION

Multimedia

The Hip, Thigh, and Knee
(The Anatomy Project Series) by D. Hastings-Nield.
This extensive CD-ROM by Parthenon Publishing Group features movie tutorials, an interactive atlas, glossary, and many other multimedia tools.

The Human 3-D
A CD-ROM released by Mega Systems that provides an interactive multimedia tour through the human body.

Web Sites

The American Heart Association
http://www.americanheart.org
Provides information on health and exercise for children and adults.

LibrarySpot.com
http://www.libraryspot.com
Encyclopedias, maps, online libraries, and other resources concerning human anatomy and other subjects.

FOR FURTHER READING

Balkwill, Fran, and Mic Ralph. *The Incredible Human Body: A Book of Discovery and Learning.* New York: Sterling Publishing, 1998.

Beckelman, Laurie. *The Human Body.* Pleasantville, NY: Reader's Digest, 2001.

Becker, Christine. *Color Anatomy! The Human Body from Head to Toe.* Los Angeles, CA: Lowell House, 1997.

Krensky, Stephen. *Bones.* New York: Random House, 1999.

Ladd, Karol. *The Glad Scientist Explores the Human Body.* Nashville, TN: Broadman & Holman Publishers, 1999.

O'Brien-Palmer, Michelle. *Watch Me Grow: Fun Ways to Learn About My Cells, Bones, Muscles, and Joints.* Chicago, IL: Chicago Review Press, 1999.

Parker, Steve. *Muscles.* Brookfield, CT: Copper Beach Books, 1997.

Silver, Donald M., and Patricia J. Wynne. *The Body Book: Easy-to-Make, Hands-on Models That Teach.* New York: Scholastic Inc., 1999.

INDEX

About the Author

Jennifer Viegas is a reporter for Discovery Channel Online News and is a feature columnist for Knight Ridder newspapers. She has worked as a journalist for ABC News and PBS. She was a contributing author for two other books and, in her spare time, enjoys tennis and other leg-moving sports.

Photo Credits

All digital images courtesy of Visible Productions, by arrangement with Anatographica, LLC.

Series Design

Claudia Carlson

Layout

Tahara Hasan